Community Helpers

Doctors

by Cari Meister

Bullfrog Books

Ideas for Parents and Teachers

Bullfrog Books let children practice reading informational text at the earliest reading levels. Repetition, familiar words, and photo labels support early readers.

Before Reading

- Discuss the cover photo. What does it tell them?

- Look at the picture glossary together. Read and discuss the words.

Read the Book

- "Walk" through the book and look at the photos. Let the child ask questions. Point out the photo labels.

- Read the book to the child, or have him or her read independently.

After Reading

- Prompt the child to think more. Ask: How is your doctor's office different from the photos in the book? What does your doctor do at a check-up?

Bullfrog Books are published by Jump!
5357 Penn Avenue South
Minneapolis, MN 55419
www.jumplibrary.com

Library of Congress Cataloging-in-Publication Data
Meister, Cari.
  Doctors / by Cari Meister.
    pages cm. -- (Bullfrog books. Community helpers)
  Audience: K to grade 3.
  Summary: "This photo-illustrated book for early readers gives examples of different things doctors do: setting broken bones, yearly check-ups, taking care of cancer patients, and more"-- Provided by publisher.
  Includes bibliographical references and index.
  ISBN 978-1-62031-074-8 (hardcover : alk. paper) -- ISBN 978-1-62496-030-7 (ebook)
  1. Physicians--Juvenile literature. 2. Medicine--Juvenile literature. I. Title.
  R690.M38 2014
  610.92--dc23
                                              2012044148

Series Editor: Rebecca Glaser
Series Designer: Ellen Huber
Book Designer: Danny Nanos

Photo Credits: All photos by Shutterstock except: Alamy, 10, 14, 23bl

Printed in the United States of America at Corporate Graphics in North Mankato, Minnesota.

5-2013 / 1003
10 9 8 7 6 5 4 3 2 1

Table of Contents

Doctors at Work 4

At the Doctor's Office 22

Picture Glossary 23

Index 24

To Learn More 24

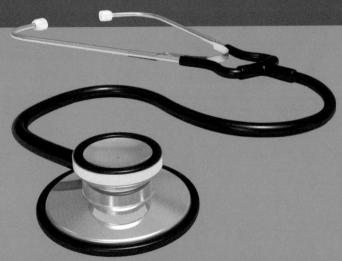

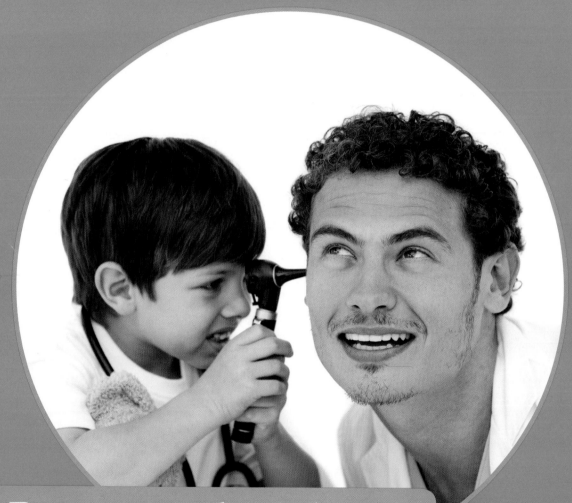

Bo wants to be a doctor.

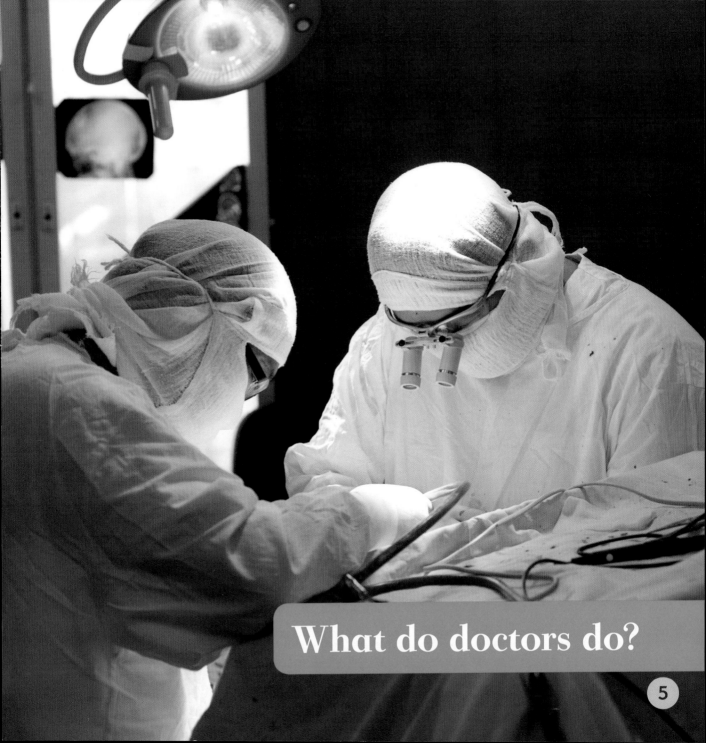

What do doctors do?

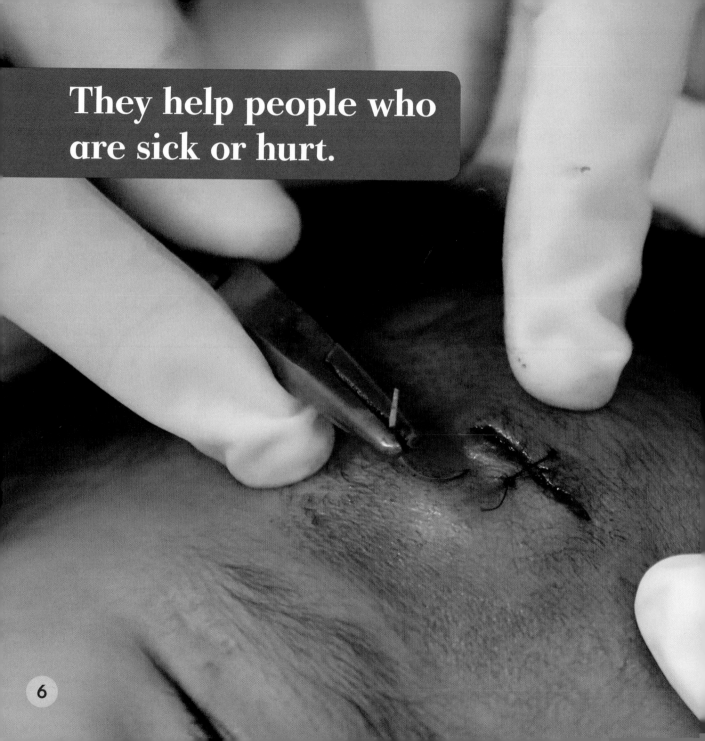

They help people who are sick or hurt.

6

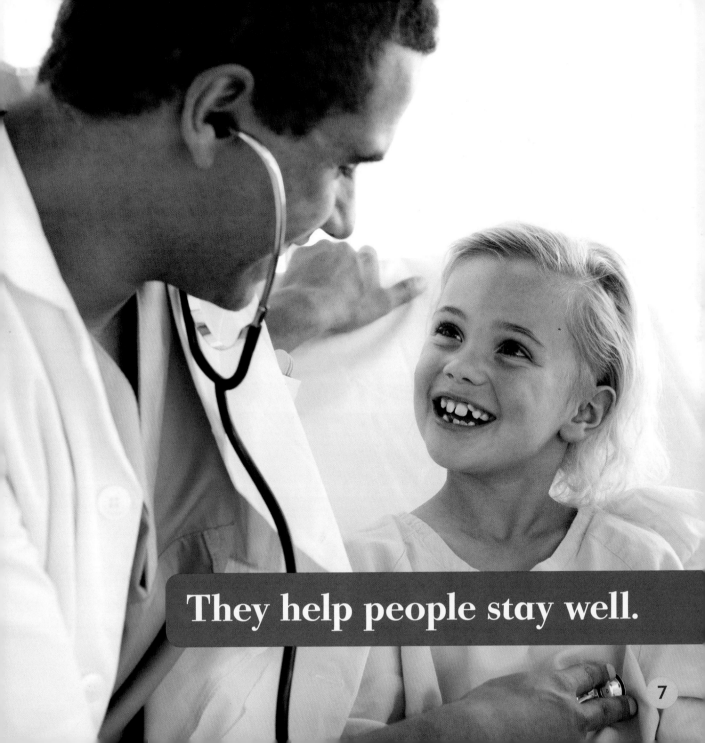

They help people stay well.

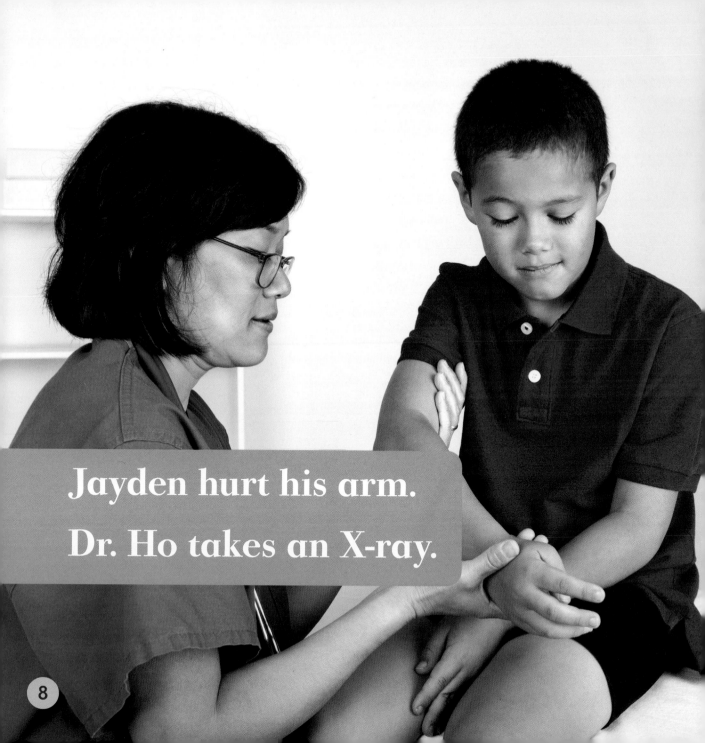

Jayden hurt his arm.
Dr. Ho takes an X-ray.

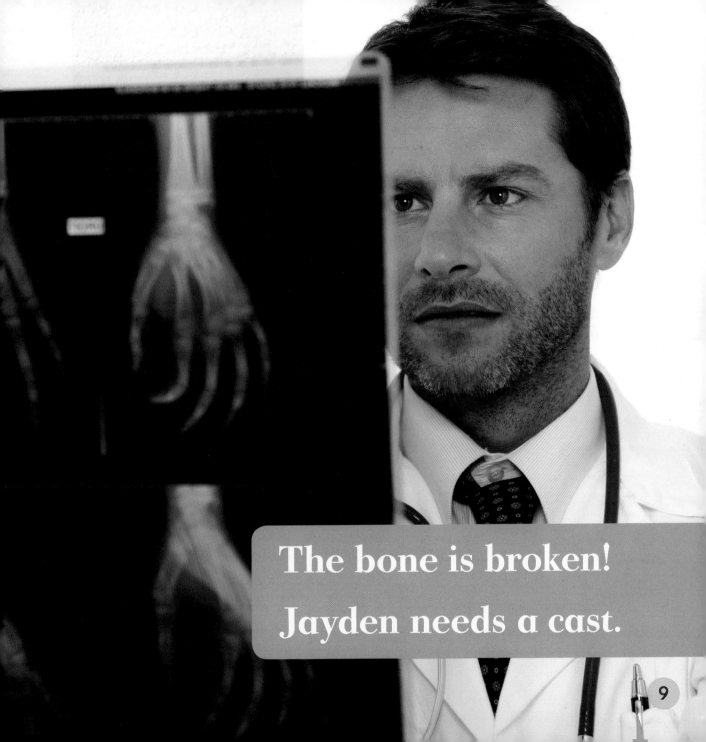

The bone is broken!
Jayden needs a cast.

Dr. Rice puts a cast on Ava's leg.

It keeps the bone in place.

Soon it will get better.

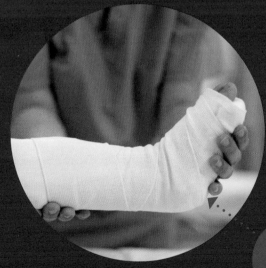

cast

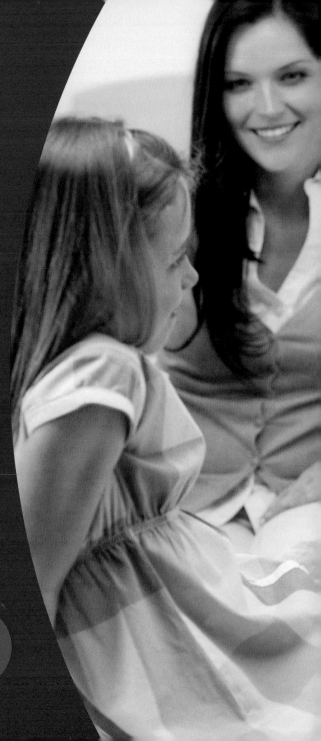

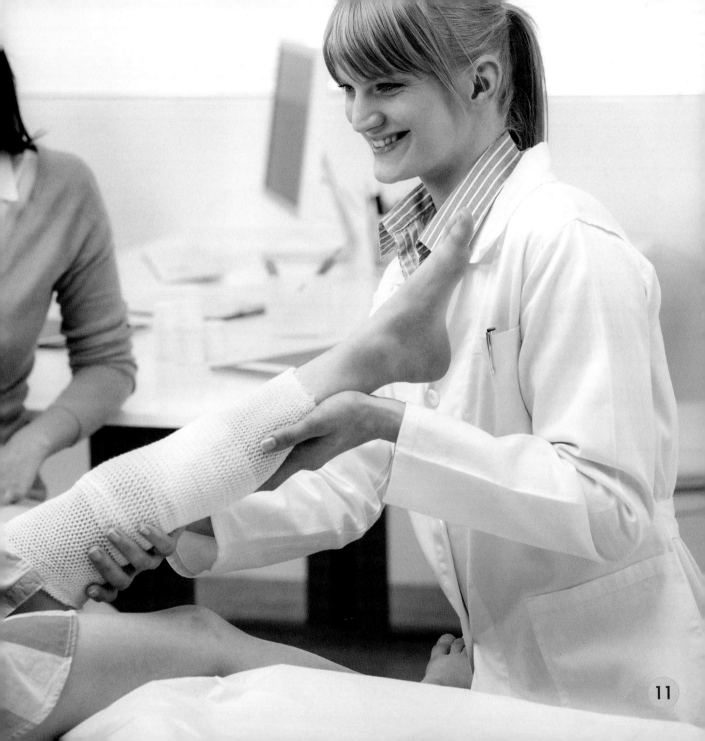

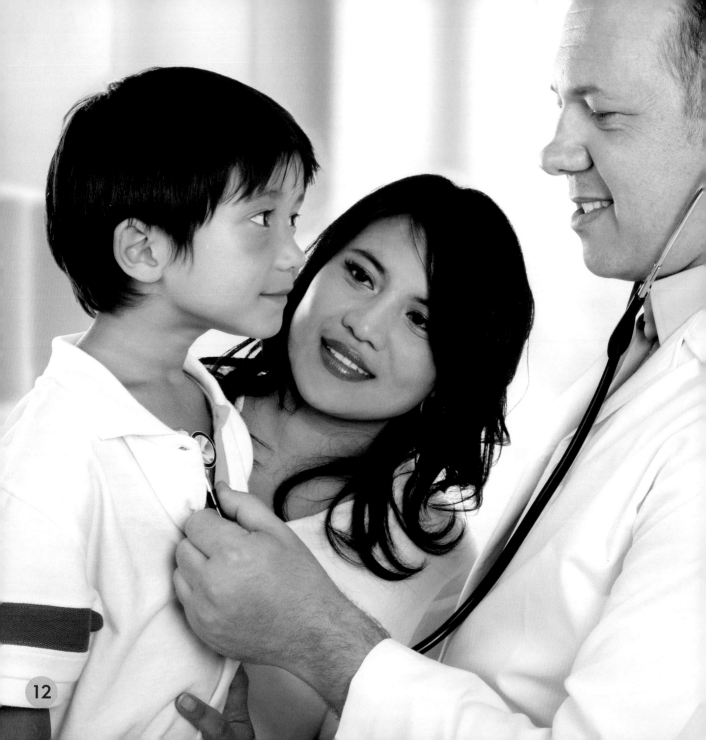

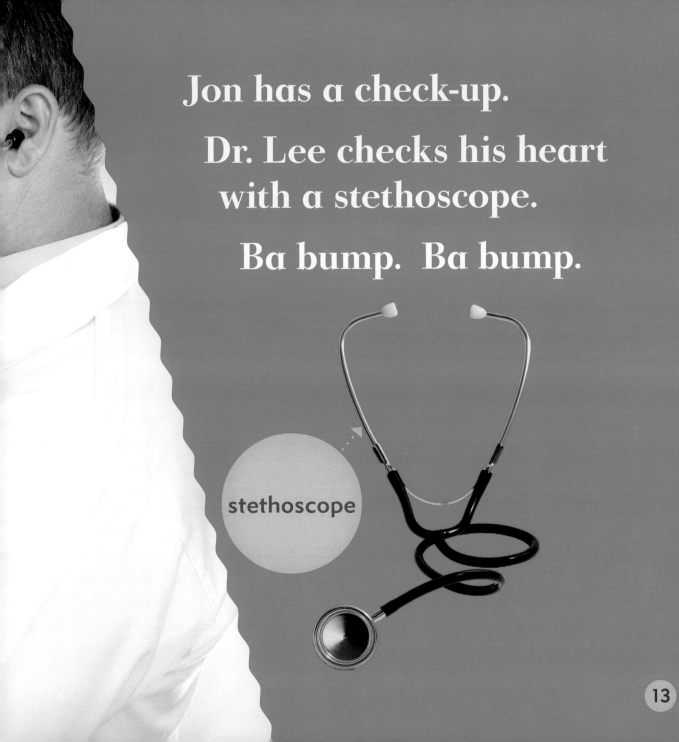

Jon has a check-up.

Dr. Lee checks his heart with a stethoscope.

Ba bump. Ba bump.

stethoscope

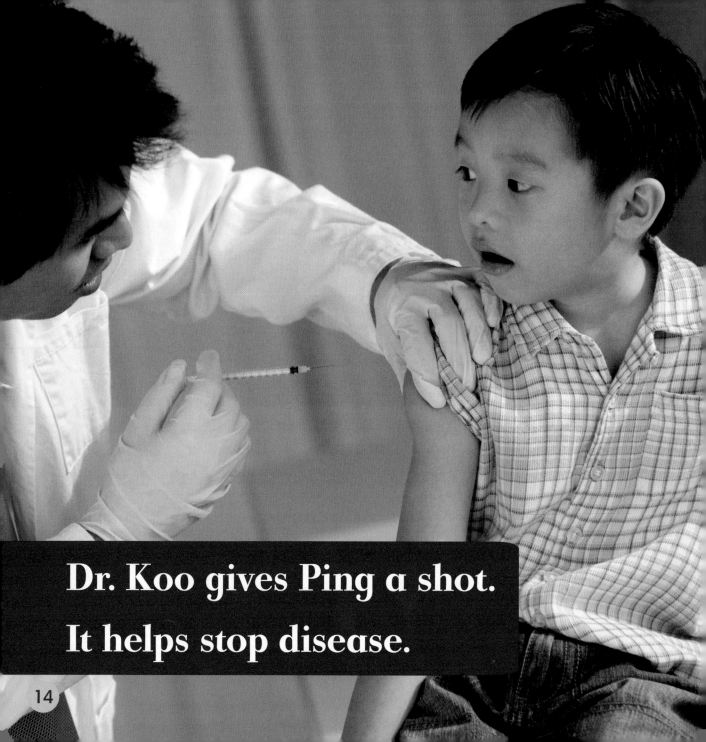

Dr. Koo gives Ping a shot.
It helps stop disease.

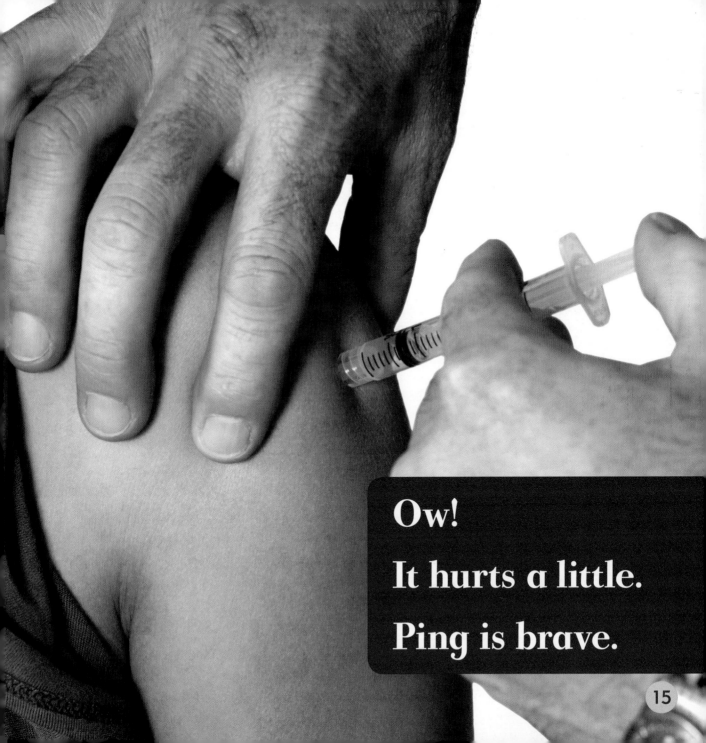

Ow!
It hurts a little.
Ping is brave.

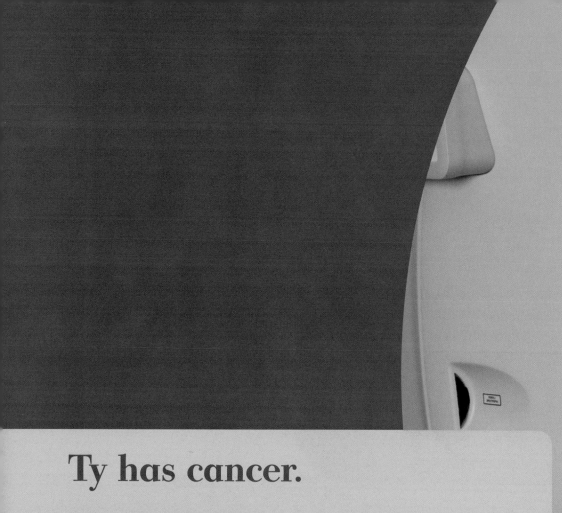

Ty has cancer.

He is in the hospital.

Dr. Cole takes care of him.

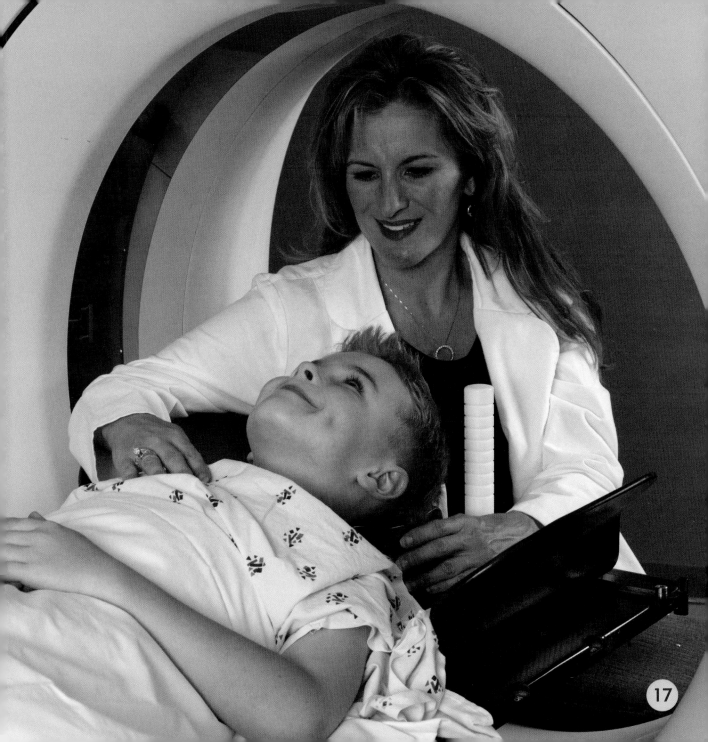

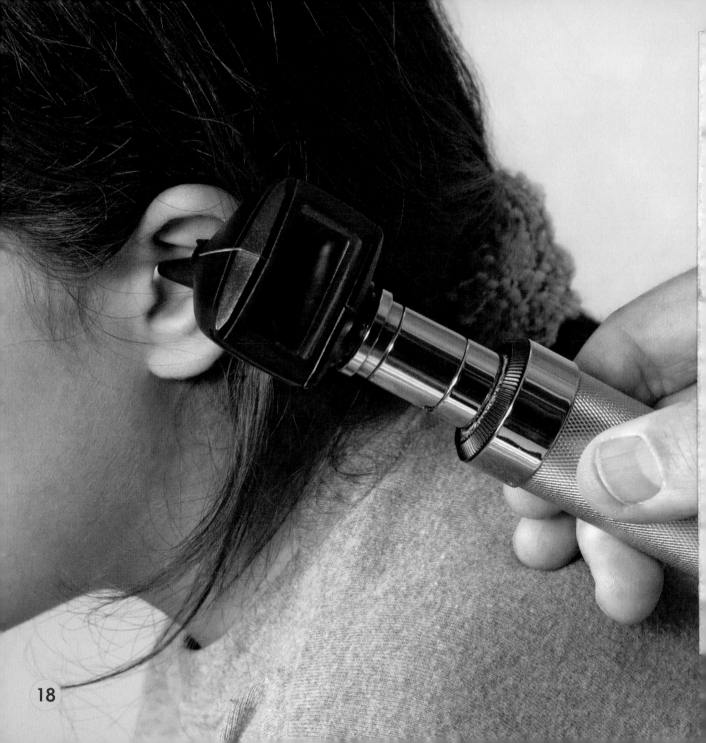

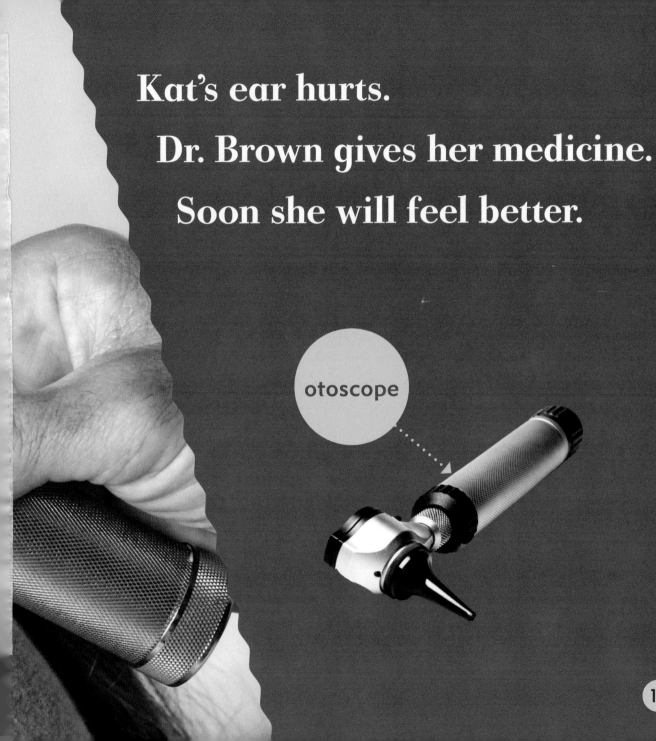

Kat's ear hurts.

Dr. Brown gives her medicine.

Soon she will feel better.

otoscope

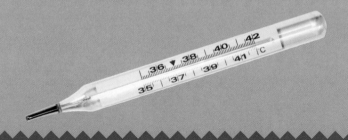

Doctors do good work!

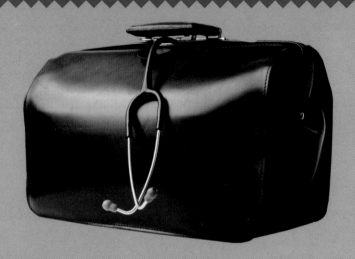

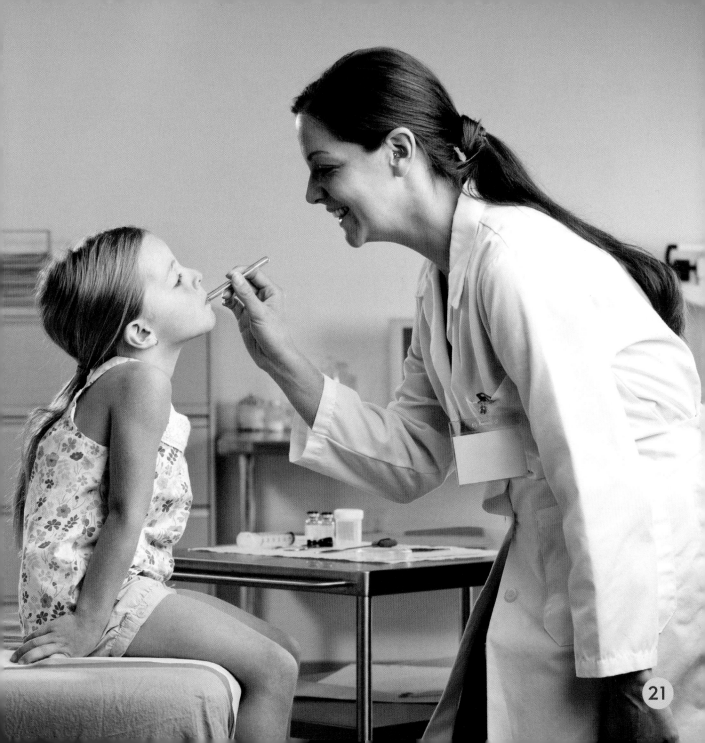

At the Doctor's Office

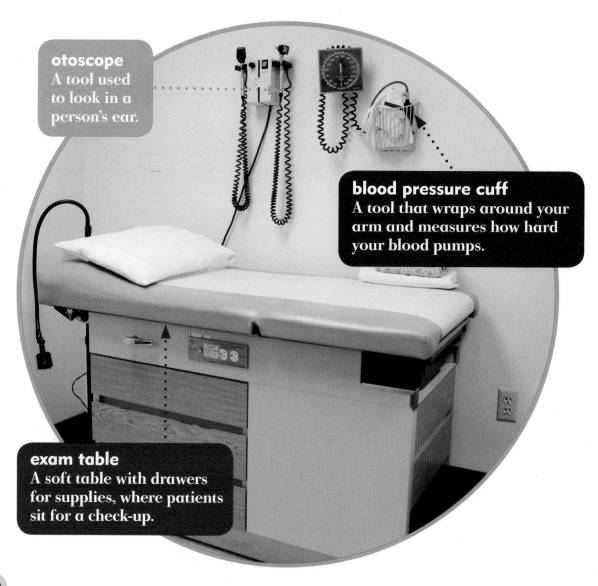

otoscope
A tool used to look in a person's ear.

blood pressure cuff
A tool that wraps around your arm and measures how hard your blood pumps.

exam table
A soft table with drawers for supplies, where patients sit for a check-up.

Picture Glossary

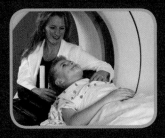

cancer
A disease in which some cells inside the body destroy healthy parts of the body.

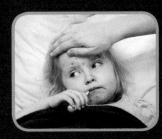

disease
A serious illness such as measles or rubella.

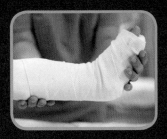

cast
A hard protective case that helps broken bones heal.

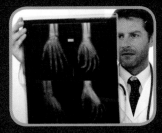

X-ray
A photograph taken by a special machine that shows bones inside the body.

Index

bones 9, 10

cancer 16

cast 9, 10

check-up 13

disease 14

ears 19

heart 13

hospital 16

medicine 19

shot 14

stethoscope 13

X-ray 8

To Learn More

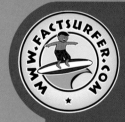

Learning more is as easy as 1, 2, 3.

1) Go to www.factsurfer.com

2) Enter "doctors" into the search box.

3) Click the "Surf" button to see a list of websites.

With factsurfer.com, finding more information is just a click away.